It's not the F&!#@%G change!

change!

Quotes from the menopause

Acknowledgements

Thank you to each and every woman who shared their menopause quotes with me. Their overwhelming desire was to make other women realise that they are not alone and hopefully give them a laugh in the process. We are none of us medical experts and this book is not a substitute for medical advice. If you are experiencing symptoms or your existing symptoms are getting worse then please make an appointment to see your doctor.

'The Change'...what the fuck is 'the change'? I hate that expression, it's like women hit a certain age, their periods stop overnight and they change into a fucking unicorn. It's not 'the change' it's the menopause and it doesn't happen in the blink of an eye. It takes a long time and it's not as easy 'the change' implies. I don't sleep well and if I do manage to sleep, I'm awake at five o'clock on the dot, my joints hurt...sometimes I feel like I've been kicked by a camel. My hair is untameable and frizzy...both on my head and on my chin. My memory is shot, I can't remember where I've put my phone when I'm speaking on it. I get anxious about the most stupid of things like putting my rubbish in the wrong recycling bin and when I do eventually get out of the house if I walk past a neighbour using a hose pipe, I have to run home to pee. My libido has fucked off and I wouldn't recognise a fanny tingle if it slapped me in the face. I get night sweats at night and hot flushes during the day...I feel like I'm a walking sauna. So no...it's not just 'the change'.

Extract from my book *'Wax Whips and My Menopausal Bits'*

Introduction

When I was at high school way back in the 1980's the menopause was never mentioned in Sex Education lessons...however I did attend a Catholic school so sex wasn't mentioned all that much either...just the basic mechanics and a warning not to do it until you had a ring on your finger or you would most certainly incur the wrath of God. The menopause was a mysterious thing referred to in hushed tones as 'the change' or 'the change of life'. If a female relative of a certain age was behaving in a strange or unusual way, she'd be 'going though the change'. It was all a bit cloak and dagger, a subject to be avoided and only talked about in hushed tones whilst huddled in a corner. The menopause was coming to us all and yet we didn't discuss it apart from the odd flippant remark about it not coming quickly enough when having a particularly painful period. I remember my Mum complaining about her symptoms for what felt like an eternity and we used to joke and groan that she was the only woman in history to be going through the menopause for that length of time...how wrong we were and how little we knew. It amazes me that the menopause has been a fact of life for women since they first walked the earth yet it's only now that we are really starting to talk openly about it. I do wonder what has stopped us...is it embarrassment, fear or the stoicism of women where we just get on with it no matter what the cost to ourselves.

The menopause is the time is a woman's life where she stops having periods and it's defined as the date twelve months after your last period...it sounds so simple doesn't it? But Mother Nature had a few tricks up her sleeve. The menopause is preceded by the perimenopause, this is the time where your ovaries start to gradually wind down and your hormone levels start to drop. It can last from months to fucking years! If you ever wondered why Eve ate the apple in the Garden of Eden, then the menopause is the answer...she knew God had stitched her up and it was an act of defiance! The time after your last period is known as post menopause and your menopause symptoms can continue for some time afterwards...it's the gift that keeps on giving. So there we have it, the three witches of the menopause...perimenopause, menopause and post menopause, cackling over a cauldron which just happens to be our minds and bodies. In the UK the average age for women going through the menopause is 51 but this is just an average and it can happen earlier or later. Some women can experience an early menopause due to medical conditions or treatment for cancer and for some women the menopause happens immediately after having a hysterectomy which includes the removal of the ovaries, this is called a surgical menopause. Unfortunately for us, the menopause is not something that can be avoided but it is something that can be managed.

When you think of the symptoms of the menopause you immediately think of hot flushes, the one symptom that has been talked about over the years and minimised as just feeling hot when in reality a cracking hot flush can make you feel like you've just descended into the bowels of hell. It's mind blowing to think that as well as the infamous hot flushes, there are over thirty symptoms of the menopause and every woman will experience them differently. Some women will have multiple symptoms, some may only have one or two and the luckiest of us may none have at all. There's no 'one size fits all' with the menopause and you must never judge yourself based on other women's experiences. The most common symptoms are...hot flushes, irregular periods, night sweats, vaginal dryness, sleep difficulties, low mood or anxiety, reduced sex drive and problems with memory and concentration (brain fog). The ladies in this book discuss the most common symptoms we face as well as some of the more unusual...you will never feel alone with your chin hair again!

So sit back, kick your sensible shoes off, open a window to get some cool air in and enjoy reading quotes on the menopause from women who are currently experiencing it or who have come out of the other side having earned their menopause stripes. The quotes are at times raw, sweary and slightly irreverent but the one thing they all have in common is they are an honest account from real women.

Hot Flushes

Hot flushes, when your body involuntarily transports you to the heart of the Sahara Desert, they are described as 'short, sudden feelings of heat which can make your skin red and sweaty'...no shit Sherlock. The menopause is the one time in our lives where we don't constantly want to put the central heating on...where the days of fighting with your partner because you want to keep it switched on are long gone, now it's them that are pleading with you to have the heating on in the winter. Hot flushes are a bit of a mystery but most research suggests that they are caused by decreased oestrogen levels causing the hypothalamus (your body's temperature control system) to behave differently. Hot flushes may come at the same time every day to the point where you could set your watch by them and sometimes they come when you are least expecting them and at the most inopportune moments but I'll let the ladies tell you all about that...

Quotes from the menopause – Hot flushes

I got into bed in the summer and my husband said "God you're hot" I replied "thank you" to which he said "no, you're really hot, go away!" I was having a hot flush.

❀

It's my own personal summer.
❀

It's like an inner radiator being switched on. A very odd sensation which makes you feel like a hot pressure cooker on the inside.
❀

I'm still hot...it just comes in flushes now.
❀

I describe my hot flushes as having a melting moment.

❀

Has someone let the sun into the house? It feels like I'm in the Bahamas.

❀

Every time I have a hot flush I look at my husband, raise my eyebrows suggestively and say "oh you make me hot."

❀

I describe my hot flushes as my thermostat being broken.

❀

My hot flushes were so horrendous that I knew that every twenty minutes almost to the second I would be covered in sweat. Immediately after a five minute long flush, I decided to jump into the shower thinking I'd have twenty minutes to enjoy it. Unfortunately I started with that strange feeling in my stomach, then the hairs on the back of my neck stood up, my eyes went fuzzy and bang...massive hot flush! The hot water added insult to injury and soon I was so hot I didn't know which way to turn. It was the middle of winter, hail and ice hit the window outside. I rushed naked to my bedroom sliding door and stood in the hail, stark naked and screaming profanities at whoever dared do this to me. Whilst at the same time shouting "ahhhhh" as the icy hail slowly cooled me down. It was at this moment I decided I needed HRT.

❀

I'd rather Lucifer's red waterfall than his piss dripping down my back every ten minutes.

❀

Is everyone hot in here or is it just me?

❀

I hit an all time low this morning when I had a hot flush...in my shins.

❀

The more women that know how hot your tits are going to get, the better.

❀

It's too fucking hot to fuck.
❀

I get so hot it feels like my boobs are going to melt.

❀

I don't drive a convertible because I've got money. I drive one because when I put the roof down my hot flushes soon fuck off.

❀

Ladies don't sweat, they glow...well if I glow any brighter I'll be seen from space.

❀

Whilst serving a customer I had a hot flush. My colleague seeing my bright red face dripping with sweat said "I think you need to step outside." I was so grateful.

❀

When I get hot at night my husband describes me as the "tenth layer of hell".

❀

Hot flushes...no I have tropical moments.

❀

My hot flushes make me feel like I'm one degree away from spontaneously combusting.

❀

I mistook my first ever hot flush for Covid.

❀

I feel like my insides are made from molten lava and the beetroot face that goes with hot flushes is an attractive addition.

❀

I was in the car with my husband when I felt myself start with a hot flush. I asked my husband if he could tell and he told me I didn't look any different. When I looked behind me the windows had steamed up...men!

❀

For my hot flushes I have a neck fan, a ceiling fan, a Dyson fan and a fanny fan all on at the same time.

❀

The last time I had a hot flush, I was sweating more than a drunk in a kebab shop.

❀

I had a hot flush just as they took my temperature to go into a coffee shop. I was refused entry because my temperature was too high and they didn't believe it was a hot flush...they thought I had Covid.

❀

My Dad was on morphine which used to make him sweat so he used a hand held fan. My Mum used to joke that he was going through the menopause to which he would say "I'm actually going through the ladystop.' Menopause...ladystop.

❀

I had a hot flush whilst sitting in the dentist's chair having treatment. I don't think she was impressed with me pushing her out of the way with one hand and ripping off my plastic apron with the other. It culminated in me falling to the floor in my haste to get off the chair so I could open the window and get myself cool.

❀

I was at work when one of my colleagues burst out laughing. My other half had messaged her to ask her to ask me if he could turn the heating on. He told her he was sitting in his hat and coat, had just had to de-ice the TV and people were knocking at the door to buy tickets for the ice rink in the kitchen...I said no.

❀

My sister is a lollipop lady and said her hot flushes keep her warm in the winter. Now that's positivity for you.

❀

I went to my GP to ask for help for my hot flushes. Whilst I was there, I had a real beauty. The GP kindly passed me a box of tissues so I could wipe my face. It was only when I got home that I realised my face was covered in bits of tissue. I'd visited two shops and stopped for a chat on the way home, nobody told me.

I had a hot flush in a department store. I was sweating like mad and my face was bright red. I must have looked a bit dodgy because the store detective followed me round for ages.

The one thing I have learned from the menopause is I can now sympathise with a microwaved chicken...cooking from the inside out is not fun.

I'm the proud owner of my very own bodily central heating system.

I had a hot flush on a three and a half hour coach journey to a football match. I was so hot but unfortunately you can't throw your clothes off when you are on a coach full of old men...although it was tempting.

I used to have a hot flush around 7pm most evenings. I would be so hot, I'd take my jumper off

and sit in my bra. When my partner's friend
wanted to visit he jokingly told him to come round
at seven as that was when I took my top off...I
wasn't impressed.

❀

Thank God for the menopause and hot flushes
because when the energy prices go up I won't be
able to afford to put the heating on.

❀

I'm hot even when the house is cold. My husband
describes it as an igloo, poor chap works outside in
the cold and can't even have the heating on when
he gets home.

❀

Night Sweats

Night sweats are the evil twin sister of hot flushes
and again they are caused by a drop in oestrogen
levels and our old friend the hypothalamus getting
confused...it's not the only one.   They creep up on
you in the comfort of your own bed causing you to
overheat, sweat and discard the covers even on the
the coldest of nights. They are particularly
annoying because unlike hot flushes where you
may get an inkling one is coming, night sweats can
strike when you are asleep and the first you know
of it is when you wake up wondering who on earth
put the heating on full blast. Lets see what the
ladies have to say about the disrupter of sleep that
is night sweats...

Quotes from the menopause – Night Sweats

My husband used to call me the 'woof' girl because that was the noise I made as I threw the quilt off during the night.

❀

My night sweats leave my bedding looking like an episode of CSI where they have drawn the outline of a body.

❀

I'd wake up drenched and would lie in bed with the window open even when there was snow on the ground. My husband would be cocooned in fleecy pyjamas and a goose down parka whilst lying in his military sleeping bag wearing a Russian style hat and earmuffs.

❀

Oh fuck, I've just wet the bed! Panic over, it was just night sweats.

❀

It was a very cold winter night but so warm inside. I woke up hot and soaking wet with sweat. I got changed and went to stand on my balcony to cool down. I made the mistake of trying to get the air circulating by flapping my arms. A neighbour thinking I was signalling for help called the police. I had a very interesting conversation with two handsome policemen when they arrived with blue lights flashing.

Night sweats are the worst. First night I had one, I actually thought I'd wet the bet. As for farting, I wasn't sure if my butt was sweaty or if I'd followed through.

Night sweats...I could have helped countries suffering from drought the amount of water that left my body.

I've no idea why I'm the size I am because I'm sure I lose 10lb in sweat nightly.

I wake up in the night in a hot sweat, then I'm too cold....I can't win.

My dogs used to fight over which of them would sleep next to me. Now, I'm so hot they fight to get away from me.

❀

We took our Granddaughter to Lapland and my menopausal night sweats would start around 10pm every night. I have vivid memories of standing outside the chalet in -16 temperatures wearing nothing but a long cotton top. I was barefoot and would watch the snow melt beneath my feet...I got some looks from passers by.

❀

I'm wet in bed but for all the wrong reasons.

❀

Instead of cuddling my other half in bed, I now push him away from me as body contact brings out the heat in me.

❀

When I wake up my face and body look like they are leaking. I describe it as that just walked out of the sea look...the one favoured by Bond girls.

❀

I'm so tired I could sleep for a week if it wasn't for the insomnia brought on by my night sweats...oh the irony.

Night sweats...I kept reducing the output for everyone else using the national grid with the amount of bedding washing I had to do.

I work in a school and during lockdown we had to test regularly. One night whilst taking my temperature I had a flush and thought it would be funny to take my temperature under my boobs as I was sweating like a nun in a cucumber field...I was so hot the fucking thing started flashing red and beeping like it was a bout to reverse into a wall.

If you are struggling with night sweats, consider changing to a wool duvet. They don't let you over-heat, they wick away moisture and for those nights when you think you are about to burst into flames, they are happily fire retardant.

I got up one morning after a particularly awful night of hot flushes and made myself a coffee...nothing unusual about that you may think. A couple of hours later I fancied another but the kettle had vanished and in its place was the milk carton...I opened the fridge and there in all its glory was the kettle.

❀

I may as well be sleeping on a water bed!

❀

I have a friend who was going through the most horrendous night sweats. Forgetting where she was (at her children's school) she said in a very loud voice "putting ice in my bra and knickers just isn't enough".

❀

If I'm not having night sweats in bed, I seem to spend the entire night farting...I'm such an attractive sleeping partner.

❀

During the winter my husband calls me his hot water bottle. At least somebody appreciates my night sweats.

❀

I keep a glass of water by my bed to drink after having a night sweat. It's so refreshing but then my sleep is disturbed later because I need to have a pee.

❀

Brain Fog

Brain fog – I came, I saw, I completely forgot what I was doing and had to retrace my steps until I remembered. Due to a decline in our old friend oestrogen and it's pal progesterone many women suffer from brain fog during the menopause. You may forget why you've gone upstairs or forget your best friends name, you may struggle to finish sentences or find the right words. It's been estimated that up to 60% of women suffer from brain fog and it impacts all aspects of their daily life from home to work. Which is why if you are affected badly it is important to access help from your GP and workplace. You do not have to suffer in silence and hopefully by reading the following quotes you won't feel quite so alone...

Quotes from the menopause – Brain fog

I thought I was losing my mind. I felt I couldn't do my job properly and left. I took a break and then returned to work successfully for another ten years...no lost marbles.

❁

I put my oven gloves on to go in the freezer, had a sweary argument with a duvet cover and put my phone in the fridge...all before lunch.

❁

We were passing the area I grew up in and as we passed a familiar building I said to my boyfriend, "that's where I learnt sign language for the blind." He found it hilarious.

❁

I pointed to some sausage rolls I'd just made and asked my other half if he would like a mince pie.

❁

My brain fog is so bad, I can't remember its called brain fog.

❁

I was on a video call on my phone to my husband when I started to get upset because I couldn't find my phone.

❀

I needed to fill my car with petrol and I was getting cross because for some reason the pump wouldn't fit properly. I carefully lined up the car to the pump and filled it up. I drove off and after a minute or so my car shuddered to a stop. I pulled over and checked my receipt. I'd put diesel in instead of unleaded. The recovery man was bemused as to how I'd done it. It shouldn't have been possible because the diesel pump doesn't fit into an unleaded car...all I can say is my aim must be good.

❀

I have taken to using hand signals when I can't remember words. My hand signal for 'bagel' had the kids rolling around the floor with laughter.

❀

I made a cup of tea and used the spoon to put the teabag in the cup and my fingers to scoop up the sugar.

❀

I may not be losing all my marbles but there's a

hole in the tin somewhere.

❀

I made a stew and buttered some bread to go with
it. I put the stew on the table and spent the next ten
minutes looking for the plate of bread...I'd put it on
top of the laundry basket.

❀

Searching frantically for my mobile phone, I ended
up dialling my number from my landline. When it
started ringing I realised it had been in my hand
the whole time.

❀

I've lost count of the times I've put the tea in the
oven, come back when it should be ready and
realised I haven't switched the oven on.

❀

I kept throwing cutlery in the bin with the
leftovers.

❀

I put a tin of peaches in the spaghetti bolognaise.

❀

My daughter asked me to get her a headache tablet as I was in the kitchen. After a few minutes she asked me where it was...I'd taken it.

My husband asked me to get him something from the supermarket. I couldn't remember the word I needed and ended up asking for tooth string instead of floss.

I had a sudden panic the other day whilst driving. Thought I'd forgotten my car keys...I was driving and they were in the ignition.

I was watching the television and no matter which buttons I pressed I couldn't increase the volume. I was convinced that my kids had broken it until they pointed out I was trying to turn the volume up with my phone not the remote.

I completely forgot the words for neutering and spaying when trying to book my cats into the vets so I ended up describing what happens instead.

When I dropped my son off at school for one of his 'A' level exams, I ended up taking him to the wrong school.

I work in a GP's surgery. I check the patient's name on my screen before I call them through for their appointment. By the time I've walked the ten seconds from reception to the waiting room, I've forgotten who I'm calling for.

I keep getting out of the car and leaving the engine running.

I'd lost my HRT tablets and after searching everywhere, I only found them when I stuck my head in the fridge to cool down and they were staring back at me.

I popped out and realised that I had forgotten my phone. I decided I would text my husband to let him know that I had left my phone on the coffee table.

Ordering online, I kept forgetting I'd added jeans to my trolley. Without looking and totally oblivious I placed the order. I don't know why I was surprised two days later when six pairs of jeans arrived.

❀

I went to visit family at Christmas and when I arrived, I realised that I'd left a Christmas present at home. They only lived around the corner so I dashed back home to pick the present up only to realise once I got there, that I'd left my keys in the pocket of my coat which I had left at my relatives house.

❀

I managed to secure a Christmas grocery delivery slot and ordered three bottles of whisky to take me over the fifty pound minimum spend. I fully intended to amend the order the week before Christmas. I completely forgot and ended up with three bottles of whisky that I had no idea what to do with.

❀

I'm getting plenty of exercise. Constantly going upstairs and forgetting the reason I went up in the first place.

❀

I lost an important set of keys at work. I spent three hours of my night shift looking for them and even went into work early the next night to carry on searching. I randomly put some files on my desk and the guy next to me spotted the keys poking out from inside one of them.

❀

I bought my Father in Law a bottle of gin for Christmas. I was super organised and bought it in September. I put it somewhere safe and as Christmas approached I realised I'd completely forgotten where I'd put it. My husband took control and told me he'd sorted his Dad's present which for some reason I took to mean, I needed to go out and buy him another bottle of gin. Having found the original bottle , Father in Law is now sorted for Father's Day and his birthday.

❀

I booked tickets for a show for myself and my family. They all arrived early at my house full of excitement. My son in law joked "wouldn't it be funny if you booked the wrong night." I suddenly had this sinking feeling and when I pulled the tickets out of my bag, to my horror I realised they were for the night before and we had missed the show.

❀

I'm a full time glasses wearer and I can't tell you how many times I've tried to moisturise my face with them still on.

❀

For some reason I put everything in the fridge...cat bowl, sugar, keys, books, phone. They all go in the fridge.

❀

I pointed out a bird to my husband. It had a worm in its beak but the word for beak simply did not exist in my menopausal brain. I ended up saying "look at that bird, it has a worm in its pointy mouth thing.

❀

Heading out for an appointment, I couldn't find my car keys. I looked in all the usual places such as the fridge and the kitchen drawers. Time was moving on so I had to give up and borrow my husband's car.

❀

I was being served in a cafe and I said "can I have a children's thingy...I mean jumper." I actually meant breakfast.

✿

I turned up the television to listen to the music during the silent part of the deaf ladies' dance on Strictly.

✿

I was standing in the school car park trying to appear normal when I realised that my son had left something in the car. At the top of my voice I shouted "Dougal, you've left your lunch." Dougal is our dog.

✿

I bumped into an old friend who I had known for over twenty years. For the life of me, I just couldn't remember her name...her husband, kids and even the dog, no problem but her name just wouldn't come to me.

✿

I told my son I was going to take him to the butchers to get a hair cut. Barbers...I meant the barbers.

✿

I frequently have my kids in stitches when I tell them I'm just going outside to hoover the lawn.

❀

I asked for a spoon for my wine, the bar person looked very confused...I meant straw.

❀

Today I managed to superglue myself to a freezer drawer.

❀

You know you've got brain fog when you bake cakes and use icing sugar instead of flour...they exploded in the oven.

❀

I went to make myself a cup of coffee. I put the coffee, filter and water in the machine and waited. When nothing happened, I thought the machine had broken...it was working absolutely fine, I had just forgotten to switch it on.

❀

I was trying to explain something to my Mum about temperatures in her new kitchen gadget. Hi and Lo became Ho and Li. Even when I paused and tried to say them slowly I still had problems.

❀

I took my son for a drive through treat and told him he needed to hurry up and decide as we were nearly at the "voice recorder thingy" "Mum don't you mean microphone?"

❀

I've been having issues with getting names muddled up. I hit a new low when I called my Mum by my own name.

❀

I was late picking the kids up from school because I spent twenty minutes looking for my shoes...they were on my feet.

❀

I regularly put my cup of tea in the cupboard or the fridge.

❀

I sprayed my hair with hairspray only to realise it was actually furniture polish

❀

I drove home from the supermarket with my shopping on the roof of the car.

I walked my five year old to school on his first day of term without seeing anyone else on the way. I messaged my friend who we usually walk with to say we'd meet her further along the road as we were running late...she replied "school doesn't start until tomorrow."

I may have forgotten why I've gone into a room but whilst I'm there, I may as well tidy up a bit.

The menopause nicked my memory.

I tried to get out of the car the other day...I was still wearing my seatbelt.

I was getting dinner ready and couldn't find the chicken. I remembered thinking "I must wash the chicken" but after that nothing...I eventually found it in the washing machine.

I went to work with a pair of tweezers attached to

my crotch. I had been plucking my chin and they had attached themselves to my fanny (ladycare) magnet...I didn't notice.

❀

I put the kettle on the doorstep for the milkman and the empty milk bottle on the stove.

❀

Remind me, write it down, set an alarm. How do I use the remote, where did I put my glasses/phone/keys? Did I turn the cooker off?

❀

I keep opening the dishwasher to check how the dinner is going.

❀

I tried to swipe the next page of a book instead of turning it...I thought I was on my Kindle.

❀

My husband asked me how my day had been. "Pretty good" I replied...it was then he asked me why my car parking cards were in the fridge.

❀

You feel like your brain has taken a holiday and forgotten to tell you.

❀

I remember my Mum and the menopause. I went to visit her one day and she wasn't wearing any trousers. She didn't remember when she had taken them off or why or even if she'd worn them to the supermarket earlier that day. Her brain fog has now completely cleared but we still aren't sure what happened to her trousers that day.

❀

My husband's boss came for dinner. Instead of asking him if I could take his jacket, I asked him if he'd like to get undressed.

❀

It's not brain fog...my brain has naffed off!

❀

I put my fridge and freezer shopping away and after I'd finished had to pop out. Whilst I was out, I realised I didn't have my purse. When I got home, I searched high and low and ended up cancelling my cards. Later on when I started to prepare tea, I went into the freezer and sitting on the frozen peas was my purse.

❀

I get brain frog, a little frog that's hopping round scrambling everything in my head.

❀

I call brain fog my CRAFT moments...Can't Remember A Fucking Thing.

❀

My rather snooty Aunt called me on Christmas Day and I said Happy Birthday...it wasn't her birthday and she didn't find it at all amusing.

❀

I was having fish for tea so popped it on a tray and into the oven. After a while I could smell burning...I had forgotten to take it out of the box.

❀

I pointed my keys at my front door and tried to open it by pressing the key fob...they were my car keys.

❀

I went into the jewellers, looked the jeweller straight in the eye and asked for my doctor's prescription.

❀

I made my husband a cup of tea and ended up
giving him the used tea bag instead of the cup.

❀

Hair, here there and everywhere

During menopause when our oestrogen and progesterone levels drop...did I tell you our hormone levels drop. It can cause our once luscious locks to become thin, dry and frizzy. When I was younger I used to hate my naturally curly hair but what I wouldn't give to see those beautiful spiral curls again rather than the untameable frizzy mop I have now...I look like a llama! It has now become clear to me why so many older women have short hair., it's so much easier. As well as the age related grey, to add insult to injury as our hair starts to thin on our head and other places it miraculously grows back on our chins...or even on our toes. Let's see what the ladies say about their menopausal hair...

Quotes from the menopause – Hair, here there and everywhere

My stray eyebrow hairs have relocated to my chin.

❁

The amount I spend on drain unblocker for the bathroom, I save at the hairdressers.

❁

What grey, sad pubes I have left, I've ripped out by giving myself an accidental Brazilian with my Tena lady.

❁

My eyebrows have migrated to my chin and now resemble a tangled web of cheese wire.

❁

My first white pube sent me over the edge...I didn't even know they were a thing. Just another strand of stress tinsel to match the tinsel on my head.

❁

I have totally grey hair on my head and a light fuzz all over my face.

❁

I'm more hairy than my husband and son put together.

❀

My husband once told me I had a dog hair on my chin. He very kindly tried to pull it off but it was attached to me.

❀

I regularly grow a luxurious shiny tache of my upper lip which my husband reckons makes me look like Super Mario.

❀

I've developed toe hair! I have to shave my big toes otherwise it looks like I have giant black widow spiders sitting on them.

❀

Menopause, when the hairs start falling out of your fanny and start growing on your chin.

❀

I have the shiniest, thickest black hair...shame it's on my top lip.

❀

I keep my tweezers in my car now instead of in the bathroom. The light outside is so much better for plucking my chin hairs.

❀

When you realise your pubes are greyer and have a bigger bald patch than an old man's head.

❀

I'm now shaving more often than my fella.

❀

I have itchy nipples and I'm starting to grow rogue beard hair.

❀

I was seriously wondering whether I should purchase some beard oil and grow a moustache I could play with.

❀

Who said men and women age differently?..we both grow beards and get hotter. Women's heat just involves a lot of sweat.

❀

My once glossy, curly hair was my pride and joy.
It's become so dry and frizzy that it resembles a
1970's minge.

❀

As my Dad got older he develop a fine pair of
bushy eyebrows. I used to call them the Bribrows
(his name was Brian). I now have my very own
pair of Bribows.

❀

Bizarrely the hair has stopped growing under my
armpits and started growing on my chin...very
strange indeed.

❀

I can grow better chin hair than my eighteen year
old son, I think he's quite jealous of my
menopausal beard growth.

❀

I used to have luscious, thick hair on my head...and
now along with everything else it's travelling
south.

❀

As a result of the menopause, I've lost hair and it's
sprouted back where I didn't want or need

it...shame you can't lose weight as easily.

❀

Shaving in the shower has become and Olympic
sport.

❀

The sun was streaming through the window today
and as I stood in front of the mirror I could see
every single hair on my chin twinkling in the
sunlight.

❀

To add insult to injury I plucked a white hair out of
my chin, not only am I growing a cracking
beard...it's an old man one!

❀

The hair on my head now resembles a dry frizzy
mop but on the bright side the hair on my legs
appears to have stopped growing.

❀

I've got a bald patch in my pubic hair...I'm
considering getting a comb over.

❀

My eyebrows have become so long, wiry and curly, I literally have pube brows.

❀

I have one random wiry black hair that grows out of the side of my ear...what the fuck is that all about?

❀

If I dye my grey hair my skin looks washed out, if I don't cover them I look like my Grandma which is not a good look.

❀

I save a fortune on shampoo as the hair on my head is already down by half.

❀

When I was younger people used to say I looked like my Mum, now I'm menopausal I've got a better beard than my Dad.

❀

I was having a bit of a lady garden tidy up using hair remover cream. I completely forgot and left it on too long...it when poker straight before leaving me bald.

✿

My hair snaps and breaks at will, I don't need to worry about split ends because the fuckers just break off.

✿

My hair is completely uncontrollable. Some days it's so wild I've started to make Einstein look coiffured.

✿

Mood Swings

Mood swings are a common symptom of the menopause the gradual decline in hormones can cause us to feel irritable, anxious, depressed and inexplicably tearful. Mother nature clearly decided we hadn't suffered enough with PMT for years so added mood swings to the menopausal stick she beats us with, we are up and down like a proverbial yo-yo, with the emotional stability of a toddler. I'm seriously considering sending myself to sit on the naughty step when I kick off. Let's see what the ladies have experienced when it comes to mood swings...

Quotes from the menopause – Mood Swings

When my Mum was going through the menopause, I walked into the living room to find her face down on the carpet with her arms wrapped around the plant pot containing her much loved rubber plant. She was sobbing and wailing "it's just not fair" because one of the leaves was damaged. I was only twelve years old at the time but clearly remember saying to her "Mam I think you need to go to the doctors because what you are doing is not reasonable."

❁

At times I thought I was possessed.

❁

My nickname at work was 'Rottweiler' as I was tenacious and my bite was even worse than my bark. One day a manager said something completely innocuous to me and I burst into tears...he's still dining out on that story.

❁

Brain fog, the occasional emotional outburst and the odd temper tantrum. I'm just one walking hormonal hazard.

❁

I say something positive to myself every day, it helps with the feelings of hopelessness.

❀

I had no idea I was menopausal. I was telling so many people to fuck off, I though I had Tourettes.

❀

I get anxious about the smallest of things and can turn something a simple as cooking dinner into a catastrophe.

❀

If I'm quiet don't ask me if I'm in a mood constantly because then I will be. If you want to avoid me getting into a mood then don't ask me why on earth I'm wearing a summer dress when it's -10 degrees outside.

❀

Aunt Flo hasn't visited since 2015 and in the first year I was really hormonal. On one occasion, my husband made a random, throwaway remark. I happened to be holding a potato at the time (I must have been cooking), the red mist descended and I lobbed the potato at him. I thankfully missed and it hit the wall splattering everywhere.

❀

I become a bit of a monster when I'm stressed but I'm quick to cool down again.

❀

The change...what into, a psycho?

❀

My brother in law took his life into his hands when he told my menopausal sister she was just going through a 'phase'.

❀

I call it the 'mentalpause'...my kids know when I'm having a 'mentalpause' moment.

❀

On one particular day, I lost my shizzle so badly that I smashed a packet of Crunchy Nut Cornflakes repeatedly against the dining room table. They went everywhere and we were finding the little fuckers for months afterwards.

❀

My poor hubby who had had to have his arm amputated was peeing me off so much that I threatened to squeeze his stump...we are still together and no, I didn't do it.

❀

When I'm not crying at dogs on TikTok, I'm
screaming at my husband for breathing too loudly
when he's asleep.

❀

I also cry at dogs on TikTok, hymns on Songs of
Praise and even some adverts.

❀

I'm possessed by a crazy lady who randomly
screams, cries and then dances around happy. All
in the space of an hour.

❀

I'm sleepy, grumpy, dopey and sneezy but very
rarely happy.

❀

I'm in the military and manage around fifty people,
my boss isn't around much and after a stressful day
I had a meeting with her. She knew I was
perimenopausal and asked whether I had thought
about using crystals for healing...did I mention I'm
in the military and that's not really our mentality.
She then went on to ask if I had thought about

meditation. My response to which was...after a stressful day dealing with incompetent men it was not meditation that was on my mind. She hasn't offered me any more helpful tips since.

❀

I feel constantly irritated, God forbid if my husband forgets to put the toilet seat down or doesn't replace the toilet roll.

❀

I can be dancing along to music, singing at the top of my voice one minute and then sobbing at a sad storyline on one of the soaps the next.

❀

I'm up and down so much I feel like Zebedee from the Magic Roundabout.

❀

I recently went through a phase where my anxiety was so bad if I went outside and spoke to someone, I felt like I was going to faint. It came to a head when our boiler packed in. When the plumber arrived I showed him upstairs and when we got to the top I felt so faint that I promptly sank to my knees at his crotch level. The poor man didn't know where to look or thought it was lucky day. I didn't wait to find out.

❀

The menopause for me has brought with it irrational and spontaneous rages. Recently my hubby was really pissing me off (I think he was breathing). We got into a lift and I turned my back on him and whispered into my mask "just shut up, shut up, shut the fuck up." Only according to him I didn't whisper it. Fortunately there was no one else in the lift but he wasn't best pleased with me.

❀

I'm like a banshee some days. It's like I'm having an out of body experience. I can hear myself but can't do anything to stop it.

❀

"What do you mean, I'm over reacting?" Said with quiet menace.

❀

I've changed from being a capable woman with a grudgeworthy memory, a sharp mind and a fluent vocabulary to being a blithering idiot with a blank canvass where my brain used to be.

❀

I was recently complaining about my mood swings and the fact that I might need to change my HRT when the person I was talking to replied "it might just be your personality"...charming!

❀

Other Symptoms

In this final chapter we look at some of the other symptoms of the menopause...of which there are many! From weight gain, to the desperate desire to pee the ladies talk honestly about farting, fanny issues and burping when you least expect it. I hope it will offer you some reassurance that you are truly not alone and we can actually talk openly about issues that may be causing us some embarrassment. It's amazing to think that as we worry about our menopausal symptoms there are millions and millions of women going through the exact same things at the exact same time. I like to think we are putting our arms around each other in a collective hug of support...

Quotes from the menopause – Other Symptoms

I have one armpit that sweats excessively and bizarrely it smell like cannabis. The amount of times I would be out and thought I could smell weed, lamenting the youth of today when all the time it was my armpit.

❀

I've got creaking bones, a leaky radiator and my exhaust backfires.

❀

My partner calls it the MAN ON PAUSE because he is.

❀

My husband has survived it too.

❀

Mama nature went bitch on me and the world fell out of my fanny.

❀

Why oh why does no one warn you that your urine will smell like cat pee, I thought I was dehydrated and kept drinking more water until learnt it was normal hormonal changes.

✿

Power surges, itchy skin and 'fanny daggers'...the last I thought you only had when you when pregnant but my GP tells me you can get them at this stage too...Menopause is a riot!

✿

Whenever I turn on a tap, I immediately need to wee.

✿

I feel like a cross between an OAP and a toddler.

✿

I've got jowls like a blood hound with the bloody whiskers to match but it's okay as long as I don't put my glasses on when I look in the mirror.

✿

Orange peel thighs? Nope they look like a bag of satsumas, net included.

✿

My sex drive is stuck in neutral

✿

Within six months of me turning fifty, I felt like my body belonged to an alien.

❀

The amount of wind I can generate could power our house.

❀

If my skin doesn't feel dry it's spottier than a hormonal teenager.

❀

My libido has done one, gone, vanished...and I'm not bothered. I would much rather have a cup of tea and a slice of cake.

❀

I think I must have sweated my tits off as they now live by my fucking knees.

❀

I have no clue what the fuck my body is going to do next.

❀

I found a website explaining the menopause to

men. I printed off a load of information and taped it to the kitchen cupboard above the kettle where my husband was sure to see it.

❀

I used to have a beautiful figure. My son's friends used to describe me as 'the one with nice legs'. Now I'm wearing elasticated trousers, long tops to hide my belly and I have legs like orange peel. But I'm still the same me with the same sense of humour. Don't let the menopause phase you, keep on being you and enjoy your body.

❀

The menopause is puberty in reverse.

❀

The things us women have to go through...I always say next time I'm coming back as a man. Although knowing my luck my dick would fall off.

❀

I gain weight by simply waking up.

❀

I've developed a spare tyre, my arse is fat and I eat things I don't like.

✿

I'm pretty sure I've hit perimenopause...I always say that my uterus has fully embraced the irregularity.

✿

Menopause I naively thought was just going to be hot flushes, moods and stopped periods. I never thought it would also involve years of the most random of symptoms.

✿

I have spent a fortune on cushions and new work chair and two pile cushions which I have named Dave and Alan all because I could not sit down. It hurt...toilet hygiene became like scrubbing your fanny with the roughest sand paper and using the exercise bike at the gym was like slamming your foof with a sledgehammer.

✿

I feel like a crusty old dowager with a fanny like the Kalahari.

✿

What is this psychoactive sorcery you have prescribed me...a question posed to my GP when he was prescribing me HRT.

❀

My nipples are back to virginal pink...I did however have to lift them up off my Buddha belly to check them.

❀

I don't know what I'm supposed to be changing into but it's not human.

❀

My farts can no longer be trusted post onion consumption.

❀

As I've gone into my menopause, the most freeing thing is the almost complete lack of fucks I have to give any more.

❀

How I feel during perimenopause..'flu-ish'. Every damn day I feel 'flu-ish'.

❀

My body has a mind of its own and my mind is out of my body.

❀

I had an appointment with a Gastroentrologist to check out my indigestion problems. I'm waiting in the waiting area and he calls my name. I get up and say hello and he holds out his arm towards me. So I happily link mine through his, as you would if you were walking down the aisle. Halfway down the corridor he says "well, this is nice but I actually extended my arm to you as an alternative Covid style handshake." God how I wished the ground would have opened and swallowed me up. On the positive side, my indigestion was nothing to worry about.

❀

I used to work in the 'organisation and methods' department of a local business and organisation was one of my strengths...not any more it would seem.

❀

I work in a nursery and when I'm farting away, everyone assumes it's the children...result!

❀

I get quite frequent indigestion and burp quite a lot...usually when I'm making an important phone call.

✿

My sex drive has stalled, it's running on empty,
parked in a corner and in the most desperate need
of a jump start.

✿

My joints can be so sore and creaky and I have to
resist the temptation to say "is it damp outside
because my knees hurt"...that would really be
taking me into 'old lady' territory, like calling
drizzle 'that rain that gets you really wet.'

✿

I have no idea what my periods are going to do
next. I can go weeks without one and then get two
on the bounce. Sometimes they are heavy,
sometimes they are light...I wish they would make
their bloody mind up (no pun intended).

✿

In addition to achy joints, a dry vag and sore
boobs, my teeth hurt...what in the name of all that
is holy is that all about?

✿

Even though I shower and use deodorant multiple
times a day I still feel like I have body odour.

❀

I get so tired and sometimes I would give anything for a granny nap in the afternoon but work, my teenagers and elderly parents tend to get in the way.

❀

Some days I feel so itchy I check the dogs to make sure they haven't got fleas.

❀

I was walking the dog and could feel the wind in my stomach starting to bubble. I looked around and there didn't appear to be anybody about so I confidently let rip with the loudest fart I think I have ever done. To my horror there was a family sitting in their front garden just behind the hedge in front of me.

❀

Menopausal Mayhem by Clare Pasquale

Where did I put my car keys?
What about the TV remote?
I keep misplacing things
Now I've lost my coat

Damn you bloody menopause
Are the hot flushes
not enough?
Now you're ruining my memory
Making me lose my stuff

Standing with freezer door open
Trying to cool my bits
Sweat is pouring from me
And I have stinky armpits

Why am I growing a tash?
I can see the hint of a beard
I've more facial hair than
most men
Now that is really weird

One minute I am crying
For no good reason at all
Then laughing like a maniac
I must be up the wall

Thank you mother nature
For dealing me this card
Had enough of women's issues
Hormones should be barred.

Thank you for reading...a quick word about me: I'm a lady, a menopausal northener and author of the best-selling sexy and hilarious 'Wax And Whips' series. For your delight and delectation please to follow the opening scenes of the first book of the 'Wax And Whips' series – 'Wax, Whips and my Hairy Bits (An Erotic Comedy of Errors)'.

CHAPTER ONE

Me

I used to love reading romance novels, nothing modern, just good old fashioned Victorian romantic literature. It was a time of innocence, the pace of life was slower, the men more charming. A time where you didn't have to conform to female stereotypes online, where you never needed to ask 'does my arse look big in this?' because everyone looked big in a bustle and no fucker was going to get a look at your arse until you had a ring one your finger. It gave me hope that there was a Mr Romance out there for us all and then suddenly it dawned on me that actually it was all a little bit dull. It took me a bit of time to realise where it was all going wrong but then it became clear. These novels lovely as they were, were missing one vital component…they didn't do cock.

My name is Ann. Not regal Anne, just plain,

boring, unexciting Ann. I often wonder how my life would have turned out if my parents had just given me that extra 'e'. I am 32 years old, no spring chicken and no stranger to the dating scene. I work in marketing which isn't as glamorous as it sounds and if I'm honest it bores the shit out of me. The search for my Mr Romance had led me to a succession of short, infuriating relationships where the sex had been no more exciting than a blow job then a quick missionary shag. I needed less Mr Romance and more Mr Uninhibited. I needed excitement, hot wax and a fucking good seeing to. I was single, more than ready to mingle and had read a shit load of Erotica so I knew exactly what I had to do in order to embark on a new sexual adventure. I wanted no strings sex. None of that emotional bollocks, just a good hard fuck and maybe a cup of coffee in the morning. I'm bored of feeling boring. I don't want to be Ann who's a good laugh. I want to be Ann who's amazing in bed. I want to be the shag that stays with you a lifetime, never bettered or forgotten.

My longest relationship had lasted nearly two years, Hayden. We met when we were both at university. I was so young and inexperienced I didn't really know what a good shag was. I lost my virginity to him after four bottles of Diamond White and maybe it was because I was pissed or maybe because he was shit, it was a completely underwhelming experience. There was no earth shaking orgasm, just the feeling something was missing and a sore fanny for a couple of days. We muddled along. Foreplay was always the same, I gave him a blow job, he tried to find my clitoris…the man needed a fucking map. Sex was nearly always missionary. I'd sneak on top whenever I could but he'd always flip me over for a quick finish. Maybe we just became too familiar with each other but when he started keeping his socks on when we had sex I knew it was time to move on. He wasn't that arsed to be honest. I think he'd started to prefer his games console to me anyway and if he could have stuck his knob in it I'm sure he would have dumped me before I dumped him. My relationship history since Hayden has been unremarkable, hence my decision to ditch the romance novels and dive head long or should that be muff long into Erotica.

I'm suppose you could say I'm reasonably pretty and my face is holding up well, which is surprising given my ten a day smoking habit, absolute love of kebabs and a probable dependency on Prosecco. My tits aren't too bad. They measure in at a respectable 36C and I'm pleased to say they are still nice and perky. My legs are long and shapely and the cellulite on my arse can be hidden with a good, supportive pair of knickers. Thongs just aren't going to happen. Sorry Erotica but negotiating with a piece of cheese wire up my arse does not do it for me whatsoever. I've been researching my subject well recently and one of the first rules when embarking on an erotic adventure seems to be that one must have a shaven haven, a freshly mown lawn, a smooth muff...I think you get the picture. I need to think carefully about how I am going to achieve my erotica ready fanny as the expression 'bearded clam' doesn't describe the half of it!

I don't fancy having my fanny flaps waxed and shaving isn't really an option as I always get a shaving rash. So the only option I've got is hair remover cream. A quick trip to the shops and it's mission accomplished, my lady garden is smothered in intimate hair remover cream. It resembles a Mr Whippy with sprinkles and I have to say it's not the most attractive look in the world. I'm staggering around like a saddle sore old cowboy but it's going to be worth it...I am Ann without an 'e' and without pubes. A bald fannied paragon of sexual liberation. That bird with the posh name in 50 shades of whatever is going to have nothing on me! Though I have to admit, the undercarriage was a bit of a nightmare and to be honest it does sting a bit. At least I don't have to wait too long and then I will be smooth, shiny and fucking burning now! Burning is not right surely? Jesus, my flaps are on fire. Give me a minute I need to jump in the shower and get this shit off.

I just spent four fucking hours in A&E. I washed the cream off and my minge was glowing red and burning like a bastard which was almost bearable until the swelling started. I could feel my lips starting to throb. They were pulsating like a rare steak. I didn't want to look down, but I knew I had to…fuck me I had testicles, just call me Johnny Big Bollocks because that is what I had. I quickly checked Dr Google and the best thing for swelling is elevation and an ice pack, so I spent the best part of half an hour with my minge in the air and a packet of frozen peas clamped between my thighs. Needless to say it had no effect at all and it became painfully clear that I was going to have to haul my now damp, swollen crotch to the hospital. Never before have I felt so humiliated, having to describe in intimate detail my problem to little Miss Smug Bitch at reception;

'So you've come to A&E today because your vagina is swollen?'

…well it's my vulva actually but let's not split pubic hairs, or try and get them off with cunting hair remover cream. Sour face huffed and puffed and eventually booked me in. I spent what felt like an eternity pacing around...I couldn't sit down, my testicles wouldn't allow it and by this time a ball bra wouldn't have gone amiss. The Doctor I saw who was absolutely gorgeous (the one time I didn't want to show an attractive man my fanny) and when he wasn't stifling a laugh couldn't have been more sympathetic. I'd had an allergic reaction and he'd prescribe me some anti-histamines which would bring the swelling down, my labia would return to their normal size and other than some skin sensitivity for a few days I would be fine . Under no circumstances was I to use hair remover cream again as next time the reaction could be even worse. Though what could be worse than the whopping set of bollocks I'd grown I don't know? So that's that. I'm going to have to go au natural. Which is fine by me, I'd rather have a hairy beaver than an angry one.

A few hours later and my muff has more or less returned to normal and other than feeling slightly itchy seems to be perfectly fine. I've crossed shaven haven off my to do list and need to carry on with my preparation. As you may have already gathered, I've got a lot of work to do. I've noticed in most of the Erotica I've read that the words penis and vagina are rarely used, so I need to practise my sexual vocabulary. I have to learn how to talk dirty…I need to do my Erotica homework. I've had another flick through some of my books and there's no way I can call my vagina 'my sex' I know strictly speaking it is but for fuck's sake…'my sex craves you', 'my sex needs your sex' it's all sounds a bit contrived if you ask me so I think I'll check out the Urban Dictionary. I've just spent a good hour trawling through and my God what an education that was. Either I'm more wet behind the ears than I thought I was or some of the things I've just read are made up, check out 'Angry Pirate'…that's not for real, is it? Once I've got over my naivety, I'm ready to try some of the new words and phrases I've learnt. I need to be all pouty lipped and doe eyed as I look in the mirror moisten my lips and purr:

'I want to suck your length'

'Do you want to drink out of my cream bucket'

'My vagina is the most magical place in the world, come inside'

What the fuck was I thinking? I can't say this shit! Firstly the doe eyed, pouty lip thing makes me look like I'm pissed and secondly I can't do this without laughing. I'm much more comfortable with 'do you fancy a pint of Guinness and a quick shag'. I quickly give my head a wobble, comfortable is boring. I'm in this for the excitement and the clit tingling thrill (see I did learn something). Maybe I'll just opt for quiet and mysterious. Let my body do the talking and my mouth do the sucking (I'm really starting to get this now). So that's the plan...my persona will be a sultry erotic goddess who doesn't say much. I'll be irresistible, a fabulous shag who doesn't want a conversation, no chat just sex.

The last part of my preparation is what on earth am I going to wear? If I'm going for the mysterious look does that mean I'm going to have to channel my inner sex goddess or does it mean I go for a prim and proper, hair up, professional look? Maybe a combination of both, tight fitting dress, hair up and glasses. Then I can do the whole taking my glasses off and flicking my hair down thing. The hair flicking thing however is a bit of an issue for me my hair is naturally curly...really curly. At university my nickname was 'pube head' which probably tells you all you need to know. I'm going to have to straighten it to within an inch of its life. From frump to fox...check me out. Today is going to be an exciting day. I'm just waiting for the postman to arrive. I've ordered some proper lingerie. I've gone for two sets initially, traditional black and racy red. Shit, should I have ordered a dildo? I forgot about a fucking dildo and candles. I forgot candles! What about a butt plug...what actually is a butt plug? I can't be erotic if I'm not dripping hot wax on him whilst pleasuring myself with a multi speed vibrating dildo...okay, so maybe not at the same time but you get my drift. Handcuffs! Shit, I'm not very good at this. He'll just have to tie me up with my big knickers.

The postman came and I swear he had a knowing glint in his eye when he asked me to sign for my delivery or maybe he just read the label on the back of the parcel...cheeky bastard. It took me a while to build up the courage but here I am. I'm standing in front of a full length mirror wearing a bright red, lacy push up bra, matching arse covering comfortable pants, a suspender belt and black stockings. I'm not sure? My tits are standing to attention and look like boiled eggs in a frilly egg cup, they are virtually dangling from my ear lobes and I'm sure you can see my minge stubble. So the new plan will be to go for subdued or even better, no lighting at all. I think it's all starting to look really erotic… bushy fanny, no filthy talking and everything done in the dark. The scene is set and I'm ready to get out there. No strings, erotic sex here I come. Well, not quite, I need to join a dating site.

I take a selfie of myself looking as sultry as possible (not doe eyed or pouty, we know that doesn't work). I decide to show a little bit of cleavage and a little bit of leg but not too much I want to leave my potential dates gagging to see more...I'm such a temptress! I've written and rewritten my profile about twenty times. It has to be just right and I think on my twenty first attempt I've finally done it:

'Flirty thirty two year old.

I work in marketing.

I like to get my head down in both the boardroom and the bedroom.

I'm looking for no strings attached fun.

Hobbies include reading, cooking and amateur dramatics.'

I know, you don't have to tell me. It's painfully shit. Hopefully they'll just look at my profile picture and to be honest at this point I don't care, I've submitted everything and I am now a fully paid up member of a dating site.

It takes a couple of hours for my phone to

eventually ping with a notification that I have a message, I'm trembling with excitement as I open it...

'You've got nice tits'

Fuck me, 'You've got nice tits' is that it? I mean it's nice he thinks I've got nice tits but I was expecting a little bit more. No, hang on he's sent a picture...it's a dick! He's sent me a picture of his dick, eww I don't think I've ever seen such a stumpy little penis. It's got a hugely bulbous bellend which looks like it's going to explode at any minute and hang on, it looks like it's winking at me...I'm never going to be able to unsee that! I quickly delete the message, when my phone pings again...It's another dick, not the same dick, this one is long, thin and veiny as fuck. Maybe I'm being too fussy, knobs aren't supposed to be attractive are they? My phone is quickly becoming a rogues gallery of ugly shlongs. I'm really starting to think maybe this wasn't a good idea, I know I said I wanted plenty of cock, but this wasn't exactly what I meant. One guy messaged me and asked me to send him a picture of my growler...I sent him a picture of my Mum's dog. After he blocked me I quickly researched the word 'growler'...who knew? Three cocks later and just as I am about to give up on the whole idea (maybe a pint of Guinness and a quick shag isn't too bad after all) I get a message from Daniel. I check out his profile and he actually looks quite fit. He's good looking, athletic and he didn't send me a dick pic. I've been chatting to Daniel over the past few days and I have to admit he sounds lovely. We seem to have quite a bit in common but I can't get carried away by our shared love of ABBA. I'm after a filthy, lustful shag, nothing more nothing less. I'm happy for him to make me come and then go. Next time he calls, I'm going to ask if he fancies going on a date, wish me luck.

Yes! He actually said yes, I am officially going on a date. Once it actually sinks in that I have a date, I start to panic. What am I going to wear, where are we going to go, will I be able to straighten my hair enough to flick it flirtatiously, how much muff stubble am I going to have?

What happens next? Buy the book and find out...available now from Amazon!

Wax, Whips and my Hairy Bits!

Printed in Great Britain
by Amazon